# COMPLETE GUIDE TO CHIROPRACTIC

## The Chiropractic Handbook: Finding Balance And Health

**TONY MICHAEL**

# Contents

# CHAPTER ONE
## Chiropractic: An Introduction

A chiropractor is a medical doctor who specializes in the treatment and prevention of musculoskeletal problems, especially those of the spine.

Chiropractors, often known as chiropractic physicians, practice drug-free, non-invasive medicine that places primary emphasis on the body's inherent recuperative capacities.

Chiropractors focus on the connection between the spinal column and the neurological system.

A misaligned or dysfunctional spine, according to chiropractors, can put a strain on the neurological system and contribute to a host of health problems.

As a result, chiropractors frequently use techniques like spinal manipulation and adjustment to help patients experience less pain, more range of motion, and better overall health and wellness.

Back pain, neck discomfort, headaches, joint pain, and musculoskeletal injuries from things like accidents, sports, and repetitive stress are all major reasons people visit a chiropractor.

In addition to adjusting the spine, chiropractors may recommend lifestyle changes such improved posture, ergonomics, diet, and exercise.

Chiropractors must complete extensive training to practice in many countries, as chiropractic is a regulated healthcare profession. They are qualified to practice chiropractic because they have earned a Doctor of Chiropractic (D.C.) degree from an approved chiropractic college or university.

Chiropractors routinely collaborate with other medical professionals to offer the most thorough care possible for their patients, despite the fact that chiropractic treatment has been shown to be safe and beneficial for the vast majority of patients.

Chiropractic care, like any other medical treatment, may or may not be right for you, therefore it is best to talk to a doctor about your options.

## Chiropractic Tenets And Guiding Principles

The chiropractic profession is guided by a set of guiding tenets and concepts. For example:

• The power of the body to heal itself: Chiropractors believe that the key to good health is facilitating the body's innate ability to repair and restore itself. Chiropractors are concerned with maximizing the body's innate capacity for healing by correcting subluxations and other spinal misalignments that interfere with this process.

• Chiropractors place special emphasis on the connection between the spinal column and the rest of the body's neurological system.

The brain and spinal cord make up the nervous system, which regulates and orchestrates every bodily process. Chiropractors hold that misalignments and dysfunctions of the spine can have far-reaching effects on health and fitness.

• Chiropractic has a holistic approach, meaning that it considers the body as a whole rather than a collection of separate parts.

When diagnosing and treating patients, chiropractors take into account more than just the patient's physical condition. They consider the whole person rather than simply the disease or its symptoms, and they work to improve health from the inside out.

• Chiropractic treatment is drug-free and non-invasive since it relies on the body's innate healing abilities rather than artificial ones.

Chiropractic therapy is characterized by manual spinal adjustments, in which chiropractors use their hands or specialized equipment to apply controlled stresses to the spine in order to realign and improve its function.

• Chiropractors in chiropractic practice place a premium on getting to know their patients and their individual health concerns and wellness objectives. Patient input and joint decision-making are prioritized in the development of individualized treatment regimens.

• Chiropractic therapy focuses heavily on both preventative measures and the promotion of general health and well-being. To help their patients stay healthy and avoid more medical problems, chiropractors may recommend changes in diet, regular exercise, and the use of ergonomic tools.

• Chiropractic care is founded on empirical facts and scientific theory. Chiropractors base their assessments and recommendations for care on a combination of clinical experience, patient preferences, and the most current scientific information.

These are some of the fundamental concepts upon which chiropractic is based. It is important to keep in mind that chiropractic is an ever-evolving discipline, with different approaches and procedures being used depending on the chiropractor's level of education and expertise.

# CHAPTER TWO
## Chiropractic Advantages

If you are looking for drug-free, non-invasive healthcare, chiropractic care may be a good option. Chiropractic treatment may provide a number of advantages.

• Pain relief, especially in the back, neck, joints, and muscles, is a typical reason people seek out chiropractic care.

Back pain, sciatica, headaches, and other musculoskeletal discomforts can often be alleviated with the use of chiropractic adjustments and other treatments performed by hand.

• Adjustments by chiropractors and other therapies can increase range of motion, flexibility, and mobility in the joints. People whose mobility is limited owing to musculoskeletal issues, injuries, or other circumstances may benefit from this.

• Improved athletic performance is a common reason why athletes visit chiropractors. Athletes may see gains in performance, injury prevention, and rehabilitation after seeing a chiropractor because of the profession's emphasis on spinal alignment, joint function, and musculoskeletal health.

• Conditions including osteoarthritis, fibromyalgia, and chronic headaches may find relief and control with chiropractic care. If you have a chronic health condition, a chiropractor can help you manage your symptoms, lessen your discomfort, and feel better.

• Chiropractic therapy can be helpful throughout pregnancy and for children who are experiencing health issues. Adjustments from a chiropractor can ease discomfort, realign the pelvis, and promote a healthy pregnancy. Conditions such as colic, ear infections, and musculoskeletal problems are all helped by chiropractic care in children.

• Chiropractic care is based on a holistic philosophy that prioritizes the patient as a whole, rather than just their symptoms. In order to help patients achieve and maintain their healthiest possible state, chiropractors may offer guidance on topics such as diet, exercise, ergonomics, and more.

• One of the main advantages of chiropractic care is that it does not involve surgery or medication. Some people prefer chiropractic therapy because it is a drug- and surgery-free alternative that emphasizes natural approaches including manual adjustments, therapeutic exercises, and other conservative practices.

It is worth noting that chiropractic care may or may not help, depending on the patient, the nature of their disease, and the chiropractor's method. The best approach to figure out if chiropractic care is right for you is to talk to a certified healthcare expert like a chiropractor.

**Spinal Anatomy And Mechanics**

The spine, which also goes by the names vertebral column or backbone, is a multifaceted structure that serves essential functions such as bearing the body's weight, shielding the spinal cord, and allowing for freedom of movement.

Vertebrae are the building blocks of the spine; these bones sit atop one another and are separated by cushions called intervertebral discs.

Let us dive deeper into the spine's anatomy and purpose:

**Spinal column anatomy:**

• There are 33 tiny bones called vertebrae that make up the spine in humans. The cervical (neck), thoracic (shoulders), lumbar (back), sacral (sacrum), and coccygeal (coccyx or tailbone) sections make up the spine. Depending on its position in the spine, each vertebra has a unique form and set of responsibilities.

• The cartilaginous discs between each pair of vertebrae serve as shock absorbers. They offer support and comfort for the back, making it more mobile and supple.

• The spinal cord is a collection of nerves that travels from the brain down the length of the spine, passing through the vertebral canal. The spinal cord is responsible for relaying nerve signals from the brain to the rest of the body in order to coordinate the body's many functions and movements.

**Spinal column functionality:**

• The spine provides structural support for the body, which enables us to stand, sit, and move in a variety of positions. Stability is increased and weight distribution is improved.

• The spinal cord is a vital component of the central nervous system, and the spine acts as a protective encasement for this vulnerable structure. The vertebrae serve as a protective wall, keeping the spinal cord safe from harm.

• The spine is built to provide for a wide range of motion and flexibility. Vertebrae are joined to one another via joints, which make it possible for the spine to bend, twist, and rotate.

• When the brain sends out nerve signals, they go down the spinal cord and out to the rest of the body. The nerves leave the spinal cord through spinal foramina and innervate the body's organs, muscles, and tissues to facilitate sensation, movement, and other bodily functions.

The spine is an essential body part because it provides structural support, shields the spinal cord, helps with mobility, and allows for nerve conduction. The state of your spine and its alignment directly affects your health and well-being.

Care for your spine with regular exercise, correct posture, ergonomic habits, and medical or chiropractic attention when necessary.

# CHAPTER THREE
## Nervous And Spinal Cord Systems

When it comes to relaying messages from the brain to the rest of the body, the spinal cord is an important component of the CNS.

The central nervous system (CNS), composed of the brain and spinal cord, controls and coordinates the body's many different systems and activities. The spinal cord is a cylindrical bundle of nerves that runs from the base of the brain all the way down to the base of the spine, where it is shielded by the vertebrae.

The spinal cord is involved in both sensory and motor signal transmission. Touch, temperature, pain, and proprioception (feeling of body position) are only few of the sensory messages that are sent from the periphery to the spinal cord and then on to the brain.

Movement and other body processes are regulated by motor signals, which are generated in the brain and sent via the spinal cord to various muscles and organs.

Each part of the spinal cord is responsible for controlling the function of a different part of the body. Spinal foramina are apertures in the vertebrae via which the 31 pairs of spinal nerves that exit the spinal cord are accessible.

The brain is connected to the rest of the body through a network of nerves that send signals to and from the muscles, organs, and skin.

Reflexes, which are involuntary responses to stimuli and do not involve conscious thought, are likewise influenced by the spinal cord.

The spinal cord is responsible for mediating reflexes, which are automatic responses to specific stimuli, such as removing a hand from a hot surface or lifting a foot off the ground after accidentally stepping on a sharp object.

The spinal cord plays an essential role in the nervous system by relaying both sensory and motor information between the brain and the rest of the body. The vertebrae of the spine shield this important organ, which controls and coordinates many body processes.

A healthy spinal cord is crucial to a person's well-being, and spinal cord injuries or disorders can have far-reaching effects on a person's nervous system.

## Vitality Of The Spine

The spine is crucial to the body's structure, protection of the spinal cord, mobility, and nerve conduction, making spinal health a top priority. Key reasons why spinal health is so important include the following:

• As a result of the structural support provided by the spine, we are able to stand, sit, and move in a variety of positions and with relative ease. Pain and discomfort can be avoided by maintaining good spinal health to avoid postural abnormalities like kyphosis, lordosis, or scoliosis.

• The spinal cord is a vulnerable network of nerves that carries messages from the brain to the rest of the body, thus it is important to keep it safe. The spinal column's protecting vertebrae shield the spinal cord from harm that could otherwise cause serious nerve damage or other neurological complications.

• The spine is built to move and bend in a wide range of positions. When your spine is healthy, you can bend, twist, and rotate without experiencing any discomfort. Reduced range of motion, muscular imbalances, and pain can result from restricted mobility or spinal misalignments.

• The spinal cord is a vital component of the nervous system, and the nerves that branch off of it provide innervation to the brain, spinal column, and other parts of the brain and body. When the spine is in good shape, the nerves can communicate as they should, leading to enhanced sensation, movement, and other bodily functions.

• To be healthy and happy all around, you need to take care of your spine. Discomfort, pain, and a generally lower quality of life can result from neglecting one's spinal health. On the other hand, taking care of your spine can prevent or lessen a number of issues affecting your muscles, nerves, and general well-being.

• Athletes, sports fans, and those who regularly engage in physical activity all benefit greatly from having a spine that is properly aligned and functioning. When your spine is in good shape, you can perform at your best, avoid injuries, and bounce back from setbacks more quickly.

• Chiropractic care and other forms of professional care, such as regular exercise and proper posture maintenance, can go a long way toward preventing spinal abnormalities and other health complications.

The state of your spine determines how well you move, how well your nerves communicate, and how happy you are. Proper care, preventative measures, and seeking professional care when needed can help keep your spine healthy and your body and brain functioning at their best.

# CHAPTER FOUR
## Typical Spinal Disorders

The health and functionality of the spine can be negatively impacted by a number of common spinal diseases. Age, injury, genetics, lifestyle, and preexisting illnesses are only some of the potential causes of these problems. Some of the most frequent spinal problems are as follows:

• Wear and tear on the intervertebral discs (the cushions between the vertebrae) as a result of aging or repeated stress causes degenerative disc disease. As a result, pain, stiffness, and decreased mobility may develop as a result of disc thinning, disc height loss, and decreased flexibility.

• The inner core of a spinal disc protrudes through the outer layer, putting pressure on adjacent nerves and producing pain, tingling, and weakness in the affected area; this ailment is also known as a slipped or ruptured disc.

• The symptoms of spinal stenosis include pain, numbness, and weakness when the spinal cord and nerves are compressed. Age-related alterations in the spine, like degenerative disc disease or osteoarthritis, are typically linked to spinal stenosis.

• When one vertebra slips forward or backward in respect to an adjacent vertebra, the result might be spondylolisthesis, a condition characterized by instability, nerve compression, and discomfort. Multiple factors, such as aging, injury, or birth defects, can lead to spondylolisthesis.

• Pain along the sciatic nerve, which travels from the buttocks to the back of each leg, is the hallmark symptom of sciatica. Pain, numbness, tingling, and weakness in the lower back, buttocks, and legs; common causes include a herniated disc or spinal stenosis.

• Scoliosis is a condition in which the spine curves abnormally to the side. It can be present at birth or develop for unknown reasons, and can affect either children or adults. Scoliosis can be painful, restrict movement, and lead to deformity in its most extreme forms.

• Degenerative joint disease such as osteoarthritis can impact the facet joints of the spine, causing discomfort, stiffness, and limited motion. Joint degeneration can occur as a result of aging, trauma, or other causes.

• Strains and sprains of the muscles and ligaments of the spine are common ailments that can result through repetitive motion, an accident, or bad posture. Pain, edema, and reduced movement are common results of muscle strains and sprains.

• Problems with your posture, such as slouching, hunching, or sitting incorrectly for long periods of time, can put undue stress on your spine's muscles and ligaments, resulting in aches and pains.

• Accidents, falls, sports injuries, and other traumatic occurrences can cause traumatic injuries to the spine, including fractures, dislocations, and sprains, which can cause extreme pain, instability, and even nerve damage.

Each person's problem is unique, so it is necessary to have a professional diagnosis and treatment from a chiropractor, orthopedic specialist, or neurologist, among others, to ensure the best possible outcome. Chiropractic care, physical therapy, pain management, dietary modifications, and even surgery are all viable choices for treating spinal disorders. Spinal diseases can be effectively managed and further issues avoided with early diagnosis and suitable treatment.

**Spinal Adjustment Procedures**

Chiropractors diagnose, treat, and manage spinal and musculoskeletal disorders using a wide range of chiropractic treatments. Chiropractors are well-versed in a variety of treatment modalities, allowing them to cater their care to each individual patient. Common chiropractic procedures include:

• One of the most common chiropractic procedures is a spinal adjustment, sometimes called a spinal manipulation or chiropractic adjustment.

To increase motion in stiff joints, decrease discomfort, and encourage healthy spinal alignment, chiropractors use a technique called "spinal manipulation," which includes administering controlled, abrupt force to individual spinal joints. Manual manipulation of the spine or the use of specialist equipment are both acceptable methods.

• Chiropractic adjustments are not the only way to relieve muscle tension, trigger points, and fascial constraints; several soft tissue methods are also used. Myofascial release, trigger point treatment, stretching, and other manual therapies that focus on relaxing and relieving pain and dysfunction in muscles, tendons, ligaments, and other soft tissues may be used.

• Mobilization is a type of passive joint movement used to promote flexibility, decrease discomfort, and enhance mobility. Without the high-velocity thrusts typically associated with spinal adjustments, normal joint function can be restored by mild procedures like rhythmic stretching and oscillatory movements.

- Herniated discs, spinal stenosis, and other disc-related diseases are often treated using flexion-distraction. Decompressing the disc, relieving pressure on the nerves, and reducing pain can all be accomplished with the use of a customized table that gently distracts and flexes the spine while the chiropractor applies manual pressure to the area.

- In the Activator Technique, a handheld instrument called an Activator is used to send low-force, regulated impulses to specific areas along the spine in a gentle and precise manner. Patients who want a gentler treatment or who have health issues that call for caution benefit greatly from this method.

• To perform a targeted, low-force adjustment on the spine, chiropractors use a special table equipped with drop pieces, known as the Thompson Technique. The approach can be altered to target certain spinal segments or disorders, and the drop pieces are made to provide a gentle and precise adjustment.

• Spinal misalignments and other abnormalities can be detected by X-rays, palpation, and other diagnostic techniques in the Gonstead Technique, a specialized form of chiropractic care. Chiropractors often use their hands to make adjustments, and each patient receives care that is uniquely suited to their requirements through a series of touches and adjustments.

• Joints in the extremities, such as the shoulder, elbow, wrist, hip, knee, and ankle, can also be adjusted by chiropractors. Getting your joints adjusted can help with dysfunction, pain, and function.

• Chiropractors may recommend rehabilitation activities to help their patients enhance their strength, flexibility, posture, and musculoskeletal function in addition to making manual adjustments. These exercises are designed to complement chiropractic care and promote long-term healing and wellbeing; they can be done in-office or as part of a home exercise program.

It is worth noting that the chiropractor's skill, the patient's health and preferences, and the treatment's intended outcomes can all influence the approach taken.

Chiropractic treatment plans are tailored to each patient and may incorporate additional methods of treatment, behavioral modifications, and self-care techniques for enhanced efficacy. When deciding which chiropractic treatments are best for you, it is always smart to talk to a professional.

# CHAPTER FIVE
## Health Promotion And Disease Prevention

Chiropractic treatment prioritizes patient wellness and preventative care. Chiropractors are well-known for their ability to alleviate pain and manage other acute disorders, but they also stress the value of regular checkups to ensure optimal health and head off any issues in the future.

Chiropractic wellness care emphasizes general health and well-being over the treatment of individual symptoms or diseases. Even in the absence of symptoms, the spine and nervous system should be checked and adjusted routinely to promote optimal health. Chiropractors think that optimal spinal and nervous system health has a direct bearing on one's vitality, immunity, and longevity.

In chiropractic, preventative maintenance entails spotting possible problems and fixing them before they worsen. Chiropractors employ a wide range of diagnostic procedures, including as X-rays, spinal examinations, and postural evaluations, to identify subluxations, joint dysfunctions, and other abnormalities before they manifest as symptoms.

The goal of chiropractic care is to help patients achieve and maintain spinal health by detecting and treating problems before they worsen.

Periodic spinal adjustments, soft tissue therapies, rehabilitative exercises, lifestyle advice, and education on appropriate posture, ergonomics, and other preventive measures may all be a part of a patient's regular chiropractic therapy for wellness and preventive maintenance.

To improve patients' overall health and wellness over the long term, chiropractors tailor treatment regimens to each person's unique set of circumstances, priorities, and way of life.

**Chiropractic wellness and preventative maintenance may provide the following benefits:**

• The likelihood of spinal misalignments and dysfunctions, which can cause pain, discomfort, and other health issues, can be reduced with regular chiropractic adjustments to preserve normal spinal alignment, mobility, and function.

• Better health and well-being are the results of a well-functioning neurological system, which includes the brain, spinal cord, and nerves. Chiropractic treatment is aimed at improving nervous system health by removing spinal limitations that could compromise nerve impulse transmission.

• Chiropractic care may reduce the likelihood of developing chronic pain, degenerative disc degeneration, and nerve impingements by identifying and treating spinal disorders at their earliest stages and encouraging regular spinal maintenance.

• Joint mobility, muscle balance, and overall musculoskeletal function can all be enhanced by chiropractic care, leading to better physical performance, fewer injuries, and a healthier, more active lifestyle.

• Better health all around: chiropractic care has been shown to help people feel less stressed, sleep better, and have stronger immune systems. Chiropractic therapy, when practiced on a regular basis, can help people have healthier, happier, and more fulfilling lives.

A trained chiropractor can help you create a wellness care and preventative maintenance plan that is tailored to your unique needs, health objectives, and way of life. Consistent chiropractic care, in addition to other preventative measures, can be an effective way to improve and maintain health over time.

### Diet And Nutrition For Spinal Health

Maintaining a healthy spine is greatly aided by proper nutrition and diet. A strong spine is supported by strong bones, powerful muscles, and ideal health, all of which can be aided by a balanced diet rich in important nutrients. Here are some important dietary and nutritional factors for spinal health:

• Strong bones, especially the vertebrae of the spine, require a diet rich in calcium and vitamin D. Dairy, leafy greens, fortified cereals, and calcium supplements are all excellent ways to receive the calcium your body needs. Sunlight, fatty fish, fortified meals, and pills are all good sources of vitamin D.

• Protein: Protein is essential for maintaining and repairing muscles, particularly those that keep your spine in place. Protein-rich foods include poultry, seafood, eggs, beans, peas, almonds, and dairy.

• Inflammation wherever in the body, including the spine, can be alleviated with the help of omega-3 fatty acids due to their anti-inflammatory qualities. Fatty fish (including salmon, mackerel, and sardines), flaxseeds, chia seeds, walnuts, and other nuts and seeds are excellent dietary sources of omega-3 fatty acids.

• Nutrients called antioxidants assist prevent cell death and damage from inflammation and oxidative stress. Berries, citrus fruits, leafy greens, and cruciferous vegetables (including broccoli, cauliflower, and Brussels sprouts) are all good sources.

• Discs in the spine operate as shock absorbers and give flexibility; keeping these discs healthy requires adequate hydration. Keeping the discs hydrated and functioning at their best can be aided by drinking water regularly throughout the day.

• Reducing Intake of Processed and Added Sugars: Inflammation, weight gain, and other health problems are all linked to the use of processed and added sugars, both of which can have a negative impact on spinal health. If you want to keep your spine in good shape, it is best to avoid or greatly reduce your consumption of processed foods, sugary drinks, and unhealthy snacks.

• Keeping Your Weight Down Excess weight increases the risk of spinal disorders such herniated discs, degenerative disc disease, and lower back discomfort. Better spinal health can be achieved by minimizing this tension through a balanced diet and regular exercise.

• To create a nutrition and diet plan tailored to your unique needs, health objectives, and dietary preferences, it is best to work with a medical practitioner or registered dietitian. The health of your spine and body as a whole can benefit from eating a varied diet rich in nutrients.

# CHAPTER SIX
## Exercise And Stretching

Maintaining a healthy spine necessitates regular exercise and stretching. A healthy spine can be supported by a lifestyle that includes regular physical activity and specific exercises aimed at increasing flexibility, strength, and posture. Some important things to keep in mind when exercising and stretching for spinal health are as follows:

• Strengthening the abdominals, back muscles, and pelvic floor through exercise helps increase spinal support and overall body stability. Planks, bridges, and birdsof-paradise are all examples of workouts that target the abdominals.

• Walking, jogging, swimming, and cycling are all examples of aerobic exercises that, when practiced on a regular basis, can aid in the improvement of cardiovascular health, maintenance of a healthy weight, and promotion of general fitness. Indirectly, this can help spinal health by lowering the likelihood of developing disorders like obesity and cardiovascular disease.

• Back, hip, hamstring, and neck stretching exercises can assist increase flexibility and decrease muscular tension, so reducing spinal pressure. Forward folds, cat-cow stretches, and neck stretches are all good examples of flexibility exercises.

• Correcting your posture is important since it can alleviate pressure on your spine and help prevent misalignment. Shoulder retractions, scapular squeezes, and chin tucks are just a few of the posture-correcting exercises and stretches that can assist improve posture and lessen the likelihood of spinal problems.

• Yoga, Pilates, and Tai Chi are examples of mind-body practices that can benefit your spine by increasing your strength, flexibility, balance, and awareness.

In addition to reducing stress, which can have negative effects on spinal health, the mind-body activities mentioned above often include components of stretching, strengthening, and posture correction.

• Large lifting and twisting should be avoided at all costs to prevent harm to the spine. Instead, large objects should be lifted with the legs, and twisting at the waist should be avoided.

In order to identify the best workout and stretching regimen for your unique needs, taking into account any preexisting spinal issues or injuries, you should speak with a trained healthcare practitioner, such as a chiropractor or physical therapist.

To prevent overexertion and injury, it is best to ease into a fitness routine gradually, working up to your desired level of intensity and length. Maintaining a healthy spine and body is possible through a combination of regular exercise, stretching, and other healthy lifestyle choices.

## Adjusting Your Posture

Maintaining spinal health requires attention to one's posture. Musculoskeletal problems can originate in the spine and spread throughout the body if poor posture is a contributing factor to spinal misalignment, muscular imbalances, and greater strain on the spine. Some advice on how to straighten up:

• Keep your back straight and your shoulders back when you are sitting or standing. Put your feet level on the ground and sit up straight. Weight should be distributed equally between the feet, and abdominal muscles should be engaged to protect the spine.

• Adjust the height of your chair, desk, and computer screen so that you may easily maintain a healthy posture while working. Make sure your feet are flat on the floor and your knees are at a 90-degree angle by using a chair with appropriate lumbar support and adjusting the height of your desk and chair.

• Take frequent rest intervals; prolonged sitting or standing is unhealthy. Every 30 minutes, get up and move about, preferably while stretching. Back and muscle strain are reduced as a result of this.

• Core muscle strength is important for spinal stability and correct posture. Focus your workouts on strengthening your core, which includes your abdominals, back, and pelvic floor. The plank, the bridge, and the pelvic tilt are all examples.

• Regular stretching can help with posture by increasing flexibility and reducing muscle tension. Maintain flexibility and avoid imbalances by routinely stretching the muscles in your chest, neck, back, and hips.

• When carrying large items, always lift with your legs and never twist at the waist. Lift using your knees instead of your back, keeping the item close to your body.

• Use postural aids: Postural aids, such as lumbar rolls or braces, can help support your back and serve as a gentle reminder to keep your posture in check.

• Maintain a careful awareness of your body and your posture at all times. Maintain proper posture by being aware of your sitting, standing, and moving habits and making any necessary adjustments.

It may take some time to form new routines and notice improvements in your posture, so be patient and consistent with your efforts. Improve your posture and spinal health with the help of a skilled healthcare expert by consulting with a chiropractor or physical therapist.

# CHAPTER SEVEN
## Strategies For Relieving Stress And Unwinding

The health of your spine is just one aspect of your body that benefits from regular stress management and relaxation practice.

Muscle tension, heightened pain sensitivity, and slouching from prolonged mental or physical stress can all have deleterious effects on spinal health. Some methods of relieving stress and unwinding that have been shown to benefit spine health are listed below.

• Relaxation techniques do not get much easier or more portable than deep breathing. Breathe in through your nose and out through your mouth, slowly and deeply. Tense muscles, especially in the back and neck, might benefit from this by being soothed and calmed.

• Tensing and relaxing various muscle groups is what is known as "progressive muscle relaxation," and it is a great way to relieve stress and calm down. First, systematically tense and relax your muscles, beginning with your toes and working your way up to your head.

The tightness in your muscles will ease and you will feel more at peace.

• Focusing nonjudgmentally on the present moment is at the heart of mindfulness meditation. By bringing your attention inward, you can learn to better manage stress and enjoy a state of deep relaxation. Body scan meditation, breath awareness meditation, and loving-kindness meditation are just a few of the numerous types of mindfulness meditation that have been shown to reduce stress and improve spinal health.

• Yoga is a mind-body practice that consists of asanas (postures), pranayama (breathing exercises), and meditative reflection on one's internal and external environments. Regular yoga practice has been linked to improved spine health because of its calming and relaxing effects.

• Regular exercise, such as brisk walking, jogging, swimming, or cycling, can help alleviate stress, boost endorphins (the body's natural feel-good chemicals), and enhance health and happiness. Strengthening and lengthening the muscles around the spine is another benefit of exercise for spinal health.

• Sleep: Getting a good night's sleep is essential for lowering stress and improving your health in general, including your spine. If you want to get better rest, it is important to develop a regular sleep schedule and construct a soothing nighttime routine.

• Adjustments to one's way of life, such as better time management, more reasonable goal-setting, and more ergonomic work practices, can have a significant impact on one's stress levels and spinal health.

Find ways to unwind that are effective for you and make them regular parts of your life. The negative effects of stress on the spine and overall health can be mitigated via the regular use of stress management and relaxation techniques, leading to improved spinal health in the long run.

Consult a trained healthcare practitioner, such as a chiropractor, for individualized assistance and recommendations if you are dealing with stress or spinal difficulties.

## Chiropractors For Children And Seniors

Chiropractic therapy has benefits for people of all ages, not just adults, and has been shown to alleviate symptoms in both children and the elderly. An Overview of Chiropractic Care for Children and the Elderly

**Chiropractic Treatment for Children:**

Chiropractors that specialize in pediatrics examine, diagnose, and treat children and adolescents for spinal health problems. Specialist pediatric chiropractors have completed post-graduate education and training specifically focused on the health and well-being of children. Spinal alignment, mobility, and healthy nervous system function are all things that pediatric chiropractic care strives to improve.

**There are a number of pediatric diseases that may benefit from chiropractic care.**

• Musculoskeletal difficulties include spinal or joint misalignments, muscle strain, and postural issues, all of which can affect children. Correcting these problems and fostering optimum musculoskeletal health can be accomplished by chiropractic adjustments, moderate spinal manipulations, and other procedures.

• Chiropractic therapy has been shown to aid in the development and growth of children. Torticollis (a disorder in which the neck muscles are tight or shortened), plagiocephaly (an abnormal shape of the head), and other developmental difficulties may be treated.

• Children who are active in sports or other physical pursuits may be susceptible to injuries that respond well to chiropractic care.

Common sports injuries can benefit from chiropractic care, including sprains, strains, and misaligned joints, and patients can also get advice on how to prevent future injuries and speed up the recovery process.

• Children's chiropractic care can also aim to boost the child's general health by assisting with their immune system, digestive system, and nervous system.

**Chiropractic Treatment for Seniors:**

Evaluation, diagnosis, and treatment of spinal health concerns in the elderly are all part of geriatric chiropractic therapy. Degenerative disc disease, spinal stenosis, and osteoarthritis are just some of the age-related musculoskeletal disorders that can arise as the spine, joints, and nervous system alter with time. Chiropractic therapy for the elderly seeks to improve spinal health and address these concerns.

**There are a number of conditions that may respond well to geriatric chiropractic care in the elderly population.**

• Joint discomfort, stiffness, reduced mobility, and degenerative disorders of the spine and joints are all symptoms of aging that a geriatric chiropractor can help alleviate.

• Common concerns in the elderly population include maintaining balance and avoiding falls. Chiropractors can offer advice and exercises to help with these issues.

• Chiropractic therapy can be an integral part of a comprehensive pain management plan for older adults suffering from chronic pain as a result of a variety of illnesses, thereby reducing suffering and enhancing quality of life.

• Optimizing nervous system function, increasing joint mobility, and bolstering healthy aging are all areas where geriatric chiropractic therapy can concentrate on boosting overall wellbeing in the elderly.

A chiropractor who has worked with children or the elderly will have a better grasp on the special care requirements of these patient demographics. Gentle procedures adapted to the patient's age and health status are sometimes used in pediatric and geriatric chiropractic care. Consultation with a qualified healthcare expert, such as a chiropractor, is recommended to establish the appropriateness and safety of chiropractic care for pediatric or geriatric patients, as is the case with any healthcare decision.

# CHAPTER EIGHT
## Musculoskeletal Alterations During Pregnancy

During pregnancy, a woman's body undergoes a number of musculoskeletal changes in order to make room for the developing fetus and get ready for labor and delivery.

Discomfort, pain, and altered posture may result from these alterations to the spine, pelvis, and other musculoskeletal tissues. Common alterations to the musculoskeletal system during pregnancy include:

• As the fetus develops, the woman's center of gravity moves forward, increasing the lumbar lordosis (the normal curvature of the lower back). The muscles and ligaments in your lower back may experience strain as a result.

• The pelvis and its supporting structures undergo major transformations in anticipation of childbirth. The hormone relaxin is secreted, hence reducing the stiffness of the pelvic ligaments and joints. Sacroiliac joint instability and pubic symphyseal discomfort are possible consequences of this.

• Pain in the lower abdomen and groin is a common symptom of pregnancy due to stretching and expansion of the round ligaments, which support the uterus.

• Postural changes: a pregnant woman's center of gravity moves forward, her lumbar lordosis increases, and her pelvis moves out of place. This can cause the pelvis to shift forward, leading to an increase in upper back curvature and rounded shoulders.

• Abdominal separation, or diastasis recti, is a common pregnancy complication that manifests as a protruding or rounded stomach. This can lead to compromised core strength and impaired postural balance.

• Increased movement, or hypermobility, of the joints is another side effect of pregnancy's hormonal shifts. Joint pain and damage are possibilities.

By encouraging healthy spinal alignment, joint mobility, and muscle balance, chiropractic therapy can assist with addressing these pregnancy-related musculoskeletal changes.

Pregnant women can benefit from chiropractic care in a number of ways, including pain relief, better posture, and musculoskeletal support. It is best to talk to a chiropractor who has experience treating pregnant patients so they can personalize treatments to each woman's unique needs.

## The Advantages Of Prenatal Chiropractic Care

Prenatal chiropractic therapy has been shown to be beneficial for mom and baby in many ways. Chiropractic therapy during pregnancy has many advantages.

• Lower back, pelvic, and hip pain are all regions that can benefit from chiropractic adjustments and other mild approaches to ease discomfort and pain. Pregnant women may find this helpful because it might ease some of the discomforts associated with the bodily changes that occur during pregnancy.

• The likelihood of breech or posterior (backward-facing) presentations, both of which can increase labor and delivery complications, can be decreased if the mother's pelvis is properly aligned.

In order to improve the likelihood of a more comfortable labor and delivery, chiropractors can employ specialized procedures like the Webster Technique to improve pelvic alignment and lessen intrauterine constraint.

• Chiropractors make adjustments to the spine to remove subluxations and improve the nervous system's ability to operate.

Since the nervous system controls many bodily functions—including immunity, organ function, and hormonal regulation—this can be beneficial to pregnant women's health and well-being as a whole.

• As the body changes throughout pregnancy, it can be difficult to keep a healthy posture. Discomfort, pain, and postural abnormalities can result from slouching. A chiropractor can help pregnant women maintain good posture by recommending certain exercises and stretches.

• Better support for the developing baby and other pelvic organs is a result of better function of the pelvic floor muscles. Improved pelvic floor muscle function with chiropractic exercises and procedures may assist pregnant women and new mothers avoid pelvic floor dysfunction like incontinence and pelvic organ prolapse.

• Supporting the body's natural ability to adjust to the physical changes of pregnancy, minimizing stress on the spine and joints, and fostering optimal nervous system function are all ways in which chiropractic care during pregnancy can aid in promoting overall health and wellness. Pregnant women may benefit from this and have a better pregnancy experience overall.

If you are pregnant and considering chiropractic care, it is best to first speak with a chiropractor who specializes in treating pregnant patients so that you can get individualized care that keeps you and your baby safe and comfortable.

# CHAPTER NINE
## Methods Of Chiropractic Care
## That Are Safe During Pregnancy

In order to accommodate the physiologic changes that occur during pregnancy, chiropractors often use gentle and safe treatments. Pregnant women often benefit from chiropractic care, which is safe because of:

• Chiropractic's Webster Technique aims to ensure the best possible pelvic alignment for the developing baby. To improve the fetal position, the pelvis is gently adjusted to release tension and correct misalignments.

• Chiropractors may use low-force treatments, such as the Activator Method or Cox Flexion-Distraction, which are characterized by slow, deliberate motions without any jarring or jarring twisting. These methods are ideal for expecting mothers because they are low-impact and will not cause any discomfort to the back or other joints.

• Massage, myofascial release, and stretching are examples of soft tissue therapies that chiropractors may use to assist relax and release tension in the muscles and soft tissues that surround the spine and other joints. Pregnant women can benefit from these methods by reducing muscle tension and stress.

• Postural exercises and stretches: Chiropractors may recommend them to expectant mothers in order to help them maintain healthy spines, muscles, and alignment. These stretches and exercises are a safe complement to chiropractic care, and they can be done in the comfort of your own home.

• As a pregnant woman's belly grows, her chiropractor may move her into a different posture to relieve strain on her abdomen. Adjustable tables, bolsters, and pillows can be used to make chiropractic care for pregnant women more comfortable and safe.

• Care tailored to the individual: Chiropractors providing prenatal care recognize that each pregnant woman has specific health problems. They will take a thorough look at your spine and nervous system health to determine the best course of action, and then treat you with gentle, effective methods.

Seek advice from a chiropractor who is knowledgeable about and skilled at treating pregnant patients before deciding to try chiropractic care on yourself. They will tailor their care to the pregnant woman's unique preferences, health history, and developmental stage of the baby. If you are experiencing any kind of discomfort or worry throughout pregnancy, do not be afraid to talk to your chiropractor about it.

**After The Baby Is Born**

Women's health and well-being greatly benefit from proper postpartum care. It includes caring for oneself physically, emotionally, and mentally after giving birth, as well as recovering and rehabilitating properly. Various musculoskeletal changes can occur during pregnancy and childbirth, and chiropractic care can address these changes and aid the body in healing and recovering after giving birth.

**Some important points about chiropractic care for new mothers are as follows:**

• Misalignments or imbalances in the spine are common during pregnancy and childbirth due to the strain placed on the back and pelvis. Adjustments performed by chiropractors have been shown to improve nervous system function, lessen discomfort, and increase range of motion by realigning the pelvis and spine.

• Urinary incontinence, pelvic pain, and other discomforts are all symptoms of weakened pelvic floor muscles, which can occur after giving birth. Pelvic floor exercises, stretches, and lifestyle suggestions may all be a part of a chiropractic treatment plan.

• Chiropractic care can aid in rehabilitation for women who have had cesarean sections (C-sections) by treating potential concerns like spinal misalignments, postural alterations, and scar tissue formation.

• Adjusting a woman's posture is important since she may have discomfort and imbalance after giving birth. Better alignment and less stress on the spine and other joints are two benefits of chiropractic care that can be achieved by identifying and correcting postural disorders.

• When it comes to nursing, chiropractors can be a great resource for first-time moms who are struggling with musculoskeletal pain or issues like posture and latch due to breastfeeding.

• The emotional and mental health of the new mother must also be considered. To help new moms deal with the emotional issues of the postpartum period, chiropractors can offer supportive care and advice on stress management, relaxation techniques, and changes to the mother's daily routine.

• Advice on what to eat after giving birth is important for the mother's health and recuperation. In order to help postpartum ladies heal and recuperate as quickly as possible, chiropractors can give them individualized nutritional advice.

Finding a chiropractor who is familiar with postpartum care and sensitive to the special issues of new mothers is essential. Follow your chiropractor's advice for safe and effective chiropractic therapy after giving birth, and always be honest about any pain, discomfort, or worries you are experiencing.

Getting the right medical care, nutrition, and emotional support after giving birth requires close collaboration with your main healthcare practitioner.

# CHAPTER TEN
## Chiropractic's Impact On Athlete Performance

Athletes can benefit greatly from chiropractic care, as it can help them maintain optimal health, avoid injuries, and reach their full athletic potential.

Chiropractors are medical professionals who specialize in the evaluation, diagnosis, and treatment of musculoskeletal disorders, many of which are experienced by sports.

To boost overall performance, they take a comprehensive approach that centers on the spine, the neurological system, and the musculoskeletal system. Some of the ways in which chiropractic therapy might improve an athlete's performance are as follows:

• Chiropractors can help athletes avoid injuries by evaluating their biomechanics, such as their posture, joint mobility, and muscle imbalances. Chiropractors can aid in injury prevention by adjusting the spine and other joints, treating soft tissue injuries, and recommending remedial exercises to strengthen weak muscles and stabilize joints.

• Improved joint mobility, flexibility, and muscle function are just a few of the ways in which chiropractic care can help athletes perform better. Chiropractors can aid athletes in improving their biomechanics, which in turn can boost their strength, power, endurance, and overall performance by correcting misalignments in the spine and other joints.

• Acute or chronic pain caused by sports-related injuries or overuse can hinder an athlete's performance and must be managed effectively.

Spinal manipulation, soft tissue therapies, and other modalities used in chiropractic care can all aid with pain management by reducing discomfort and facilitating recovery.

• Chiropractors can help injured athletes get back in the game by prescribing rehabilitation exercises, stretches, and other therapies that speed up the healing process, restore function, and reduce the risk of further injury.

Chiropractic care can be used in conjunction with other rehabilitation methods, such as physical therapy, to speed up and improve the quality of an athlete's return to play.

• Chiropractic care also includes advice on nutrition, hydration, and lifestyle choices that can improve an athlete's performance and speed up their recovery time. Athletes' health and performance can benefit from advice on ergonomics, sleep, and stress management.

• Different athletes have different needs, therefore chiropractors can modify treatment regimens accordingly. Athletes receive individualized care that is tailored to their specific sport, training schedule, injury history, and other concerns.

• Chiropractic therapy for athletes is often provided in conjunction with other medical professionals, such as sports medicine doctors, physical therapists, and even coaches. By working together, doctors of chiropractic can better help athletes in terms of their overall health and performance.

Athletes should seek out chiropractors who have experience

and skill in sports chiropractic, and the chiropractic care they receive should be based on solid scientific data. In order to receive the most beneficial and risk-free chiropractic therapy for sports performance, athletes should be open and honest with their healthcare team about their individual needs, goals, and concerns.

## Chiropractors Who Specialize On Sports Injuries

Sports chiropractors often adapt their methods to meet the unique demands of each sport and participant. Some of the most popular chiropractic procedures utilized in sports are as follows:

• Chiropractors employ a variety of procedures, including manual and instrument-assisted adjustments, to restore joint mobility and alignment. This can aid in increasing range of motion in the joints, decreasing muscle imbalances, and enhancing biomechanics for peak athletic performance.

• Myofascial release, trigger point therapy, and instrument-assisted soft tissue mobilization (IASTM) are examples of soft tissue therapies used by chiropractors to treat muscle imbalances, alleviate muscle tension, and speed up the healing process. Tight muscles, overuse injuries, and post-workout fatigue can all be alleviated with these methods.

• Specific rehabilitation activities may be prescribed by chiropractors for athletes based on their sport and individual demands. Strength, flexibility, stability, and coordination are all important for sports performance and injury prevention, and can be enhanced with these activities.

• Kinesiology tape is often used by chiropractors to help stabilize and protect injured or weak areas while also reducing associated discomfort. Athletes can benefit from kinesiology tape since it aids in muscle function and biomechanics.

• Chiropractors can help athletes reach their full potential by using procedures developed specifically for the purpose of improving their performance in a given sport. Techniques that target hip and knee alignment, for instance, may be helpful for runners, while those that target spine rotation and mobility may be helpful for golfers.

• Chiropractors may employ functional movement evaluations to evaluate an athlete's movement patterns and detect any imbalances or dysfunctions that could negatively affect the athlete's ability to perform in their chosen sport.

Chiropractors might use assessment data to tailor treatment strategies to address specific complaints and boost patients' functional mobility.

• Chiropractors can help athletes improve their performance, energy, and recuperation by advising them on proper sports nutrition and hydration.

Based on the athlete's sport, training schedule, and individual demands, they may suggest solutions for proper nutritional intake, hydration, and supplementation.

It is worth noting that specific chiropractic treatments used in sports chiropractic may differ from patient to patient and from sport to sport. Sports chiropractors understand that each athlete is different and will modify their treatment accordingly, all while collaborating closely with other medical professionals.

# CHAPTER ELEVEN
## Chiropractic Ethics And Professionalism

As in other medical fields, chiropractic therapy is conducted with the utmost professionalism and adherence to ethical standards.

There is a strict code of ethics that chiropractors must follow to provide their patients with the best possible care. Some foundational principles of chiropractic professionalism and ethics are as follows:

• Chiropractic therapy is patient-centered because chiropractors have an ethical obligation to look out for their patients' best interests first and foremost. Maintaining a trustworthy, honest, and mutually respectful professional relationship with patients entails adhering to these principles.

• Maintaining a high level of competency in practice is the responsibility of chiropractors, and they can do so by regular participation in continuing education programs and other forms of professional development. This guarantees that they are familiar with the most recent discoveries, methods, and standards in chiropractic care.

• Boundaries in the workplace Chiropractors are expected to avoid any activity that could jeopardize the therapeutic relationship with their patients, including conflicts of interest, dual relationships, and other potentially harmful situations. They also should not get involved in anything dishonest or illegal.

- Honesty and integrity Chiropractors should always treat their patients, coworkers, and the general public with the utmost honesty and integrity. They should be truthful about their experience, training, and the results you can expect from treatment, and they should never make false or exaggerated claims.

- Chiropractors should treat each patient with dignity and respect, taking into account their unique history, lifestyle, and cultural background. Every patient deserves treatment that respects their individuality and dignity and is free from bias and prejudice.

• Chiropractors, like other healthcare professionals, should work together for the benefit of their patients and take part in interdisciplinary care as necessary. This involves working as part of a healthcare team, which involves communicating effectively with other professionals in the field, sending patients to the appropriate specialists when necessary, and so on.

• Chiropractors are expected to uphold the chiropractic profession's reputation by their professional demeanor and appearance. You must present yourself in a professional manner at all times, treating patients, coworkers, and staff with the utmost respect and courtesy.

• Chiropractors must follow all applicable rules, regulations, and guidelines governing the chiropractic profession, such as those pertaining to license, scope of practice, documentation, billing, and insurance. They should also be conversant with the ethical rules and standards established by their regulatory organizations or professional groups in the field of chiropractic.

• Safeguarding patient information and records in compliance with existing rules and regulations and only revealing patient information with appropriate consent or as required by law are two ways in which chiropractors show respect for their patients' right to privacy and confidentiality.

• Self-reflection and professional responsibility: Chiropractors need to own up to their mistakes, examine their methods, and always work to become better at what they do.

They must be receptive to criticism, seek out direction when they are unsure of what to do, and deal with any ethical conflicts or issues in a timely fashion.

A chiropractor's ability to deliver safe, effective, and compassionate care, as well as to preserve the trust and confidence of patients, colleagues, and the public, hinges on his or her adherence to the principles of ethics and professionalism.

## Establishing A Prosperous Chiropractic Clinic

Establishing a thriving chiropractic office calls for a unique blend of clinical knowledge, financial savvy, and attention to individual patients. You may build a successful chiropractic practice by following these guidelines.

• First, you should establish your goals for your chiropractic clinic and write out a detailed business strategy. Your vision, objectives, target demographic, proposed methods of reaching them, projected revenues, and future expansion plans all belong here.

• Create a memorable brand identity for your chiropractic clinic by developing a memorable name, logo, and website. Professional website design, search engine optimization (SEO), and social media marketing are all essential in today's digital world if you want to attract and keep patients.

• Focus on providing excellent treatment to patients and making their stay as pleasant as possible. Establish trust with patients, address their issues, create individualized treatment programs, and make sure they are always happy and relaxed under your care as a chiropractor.

• Create successful advertising campaigns: use focused advertising to find and keep patients. Online and social media marketing, public relations, patient referrals, and collaboration with other businesses and medical professionals in the area are all possibilities.

• Provide outstanding service at every stage of the patient's interaction with your practice, from the initial phone call or email enquiry through appointment scheduling, check-in, and any necessary follow-up care. Patient satisfaction that results in positive word-of-mouth referrals is a major growth engine.

• Do outreach work in your neighborhood by attending and assisting with community activities like health fairs and workshops.

By doing so, you can promote chiropractic care, solidify your reputation as a reliable healthcare practitioner, and network with others who may benefit from your services.

• If you want to improve productivity and efficiency, it is important to use sound practice management techniques. Appointment management software, electronic health records (EHRs), billing and coding procedures, and well-trained employees can all contribute to a well-run medical practice.

• Grow your referral base by networking with other professionals in the medical field. This includes physicians, physiotherapists, and athletic trainers. Working with other experts can boost your reputation and bring in more patients who need specialized care.

• Spend time and money on training and education to improve your skills as a chiropractor and provide the finest care possible for your patients. Improve your clinical abilities and expertise by furthering your education in conferences, workshops, and seminars.

• The success of a practice depends heavily on the retention of current patients. Think of ways to keep your patients interested, well-informed, and content throughout their treatment. The patient may be educated, spoken with, followed up on, and have any issues or concerns addressed proactively as part of this.

• Track your progress toward your business goals by regularly monitoring and measuring your practice's performance against key performance indicators (KPIs).

Retention rates, acquisition rates, revenue, expenses, and patient satisfaction surveys are all examples. Make better judgments and pinpoint problem areas to boost your practice's efficiency with the help of this data.

Establishing a thriving chiropractic clinic is a labor of love that requires time, energy, and commitment. You can build a successful chiropractic practice that serves your patients' needs and contributes to your professional success if you focus on providing exceptional patient care, implementing effective marketing strategies, cultivating professional relationships, and continuously improving your clinical and business skills.

## Conclusion

Chiropractic is a form of alternative medicine that takes a more integrative and natural approach to patient care by looking at the whole person rather than just the symptoms.

In this field, the spine plays a central role in the diagnosis, treatment, and prevention of musculoskeletal diseases. Chiropractors use a wide range of manual therapies to aid patients in restoring and maintaining spinal health, reducing pain and restoring function.

We have covered a lot of ground in this book, from chiropractic's guiding principles and philosophy to its advantages and techniques to its applications across the lifespan (from pediatrics to geriatrics to pregnancy to athletic performance).

We also talked about how chiropractic care might benefit from attention to things like diet, exercise, posture, stress reduction, and professional conduct.

Establishing a thriving chiropractic office calls for a unique blend of clinical knowledge, financial savvy, and attention to individual patients.

Chiropractors can achieve success in their careers and meet the needs of their patients by providing excellent care to their patients, utilizing successful marketing strategies, building strong professional relationships, and regularly updating their clinical and business knowledge.

Chiropractic is an all-natural, drug-free, and holistic method of treatment that primarily targets the spine and nervous system in an effort to improve general health and well-being.

It has been proven useful for a variety of musculoskeletal disorders, as well as for general wellness and preventative medicine. An individual's health care regimen may benefit from chiropractic treatment, and chiropractors play an important role in assisting their patients in achieving and maintaining optimal spinal health and well-being.

# THE END